Skin Health Cuisine

A Cookbook for Shingles and Psoriasis Warriors.

BY

Kellie V. Ross

Copyright

Radiance: Sarah's Journey to Healing with Skin Health Cuisine

In a small town nestled between rolling hills, lived a woman named Sarah. Sarah was a warrior, but not of the kind you read about in epic tales. She was a warrior battling an invisible foe psoriasis. Her journey was one of courage, resilience, and ultimately, triumph, and it all began when she discovered **"Skin Health Cuisine: A Cookbook for Shingles and Psoriasis Warriors."**

Sarah's life had been a constant struggle. Psoriasis had taken its toll on her skin, leaving her feeling self-conscious and burdened. The relentless itching and discomfort were her constant companions. She'd tried numerous treatments, but nothing seemed to provide the relief she so desperately sought.

One gloomy afternoon, Sarah's friend Emma, who had witnessed her struggles, visited with a gift in hand. It was a cookbook. "I heard about this cookbook," Emma said, "and I thought it might help you. It's called **"Skin Health Cuisine"**.

Sarah's heart skipped a beat. Could this be the answer she had been searching for? She flipped through the pages and saw the tantalizing recipes, each one carefully crafted to support skin health. She read about the healing power of antioxidants, the benefits of omega-3 fatty acids, and the soothing properties of certain herbs.

Determined to take control of her health, Sarah embarked on a journey with the cookbook as her guide. She started her day with a vibrant blueberry smoothie, savoring each sip, knowing that every antioxidant-packed berry was nourishing her skin from within. She followed the cookbook's meal plans religiously, each day bringing a new culinary adventure.

As she explored the world of skin-nourishing cuisine, Sarah felt a profound transformation within herself. The chronic itching began to subside, and her skin started to regain its natural glow. She could hardly believe it. For the first time in years, she was finding relief, not in expensive medications, but in the very food she put on her plate.

But the cookbook offered more than just recipes. It provided guidance on managing stress, nurturing mental health, and building a support network. Sarah learned the power of self-compassion and the importance of self-care. She started practicing yoga and meditation, finding solace in these moments of tranquility.

Sarah's journey wasn't without challenges. There were days when her skin still flared up, reminding her that healing is not always linear. But she had discovered a resilience within herself, a warrior spirit that refused to be defeated. She continued to cook, to savor, and to nurture herself.

Months turned into years, and as Sarah continued her journey with "Skin Health Cuisine," she not only reclaimed her skin but also her confidence. She stepped out into the world with a newfound radiance, a testament to the healing power of food, self-love, and unwavering determination.

One day, while shopping for groceries, Sarah bumped into Emma, the friend who had introduced her to the cookbook that had changed her life. Tears welled up in her eyes as she hugged Emma tightly. "You saved me," she whispered. "You gave me the gift of healing."

Emma smiled, her heart warmed by Sarah's transformation. "No, my dear," she said, "you saved yourself. You are the true warrior in this story. I just handed you the sword."

Sarah's story is one of triumph over adversity, a testament to the power of self-care and the healing potential that lies in the food we eat. She is a living embodiment of the strength that resides within each of us, waiting to be awakened by the right knowledge, the right choices, and the right cookbook.

TABLE OF CONTENTS

INTRODUCTION

"Are you tired of feeling like your skin is waging a constant battle against discomfort and irritation? Does the frustration of dealing with shingles or psoriasis sometimes make you want to scream? If you've ever found yourself in these moments of exasperation, you're not alone.

Living with skin conditions like shingles and psoriasis can be emotionally and physically taxing. The itching, the discomfort, and the self-consciousness can take a toll on your well-being. But there's hope, and it comes in the form of **"Skin Health Cuisine: A Cookbook for Shingles and Psoriasis Warriors."**

This cookbook isn't just about recipes; it's a lifeline for those who refuse to be defined by their skin conditions. It's a celebration of your resilience, your determination, and your commitment to living your best life, even in the face of these challenges.

In a world where taking care of your skin can feel like an uphill battle, this cookbook is your trusted companion. It's a guide to understanding the healing power of food, the importance of self-care, and the joy of savoring every bite. With recipes designed to nourish your skin from the inside out, you'll discover that food can be your ally in this journey.

As you explore the pages ahead, you'll find not only delicious recipes but also insights into controlling discomfort, managing flare-ups, and nurturing your skin's well-being. Whether you're dealing with shingles, psoriasis, or both, this book is your roadmap to healthier, happier skin.

So, if you're ready to embark on a journey of self-care, healing, and embracing your inner warrior, let **"Skin Health Cuisine"** be your guide. It's not just a cookbook; it's your ticket to a more radiant and resilient you.

RECIPE 1:

Blueberry Bliss Smoothie

Total Time: Approximately 10 minutes

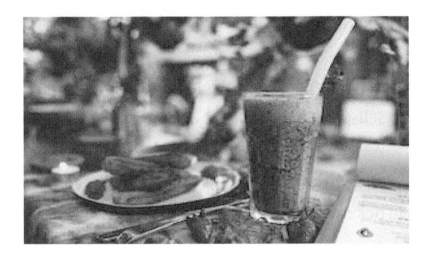

Ingredients:

- 1 cup fresh or frozen blueberries
- 1/2 ripe avocado

- 1/2 cup Greek yogurt (or dairy-free alternative)
- 1 tablespoon honey (optional)
- 1/2 cup spinach leaves
- 1/2 cup unsweetened almond milk (or your preferred milk)
- 1/2 teaspoon ground turmeric (for its anti-inflammatory properties)
- Ice cubes (optional)

Instructions:

1. *Preparation (2 minutes):* Gather all your ingredients and equipment.

2. *Blend (3 minutes):* In a blender, combine the blueberries, ripe avocado, Greek yogurt

(or dairy-free alternative), and honey if desired. These ingredients are packed with antioxidants and healthy fats to support your skin.

3. *Add Spinach (1 minute):* Add the spinach leaves for an extra boost of vitamins and minerals. Spinach is known for its skin-brightening properties.

4. *Pour Milk (1 minute):* Pour in the unsweetened almond milk, which is hydrating and gentle on the skin.

5. *Turmeric (1 minute):* To harness the anti-inflammatory benefits of turmeric, sprinkle in the ground turmeric.

6. *Blend Again (2 minutes):* If you prefer a colder smoothie, add some ice cubes to the blender. Then, blend all the ingredients until smooth and creamy.

7. *Taste and Adjust (1 minute):* Taste the smoothie and adjust the sweetness with more honey if needed.

8. *Serve (1 minute):* Pour your Blueberry Bliss Smoothie into a glass, garnish with a few fresh blueberries, and enjoy the nourishing goodness!

RECIPE 2:

Baked Salmon with Lemon and Dill

Total Time: Approximately 30 minutes

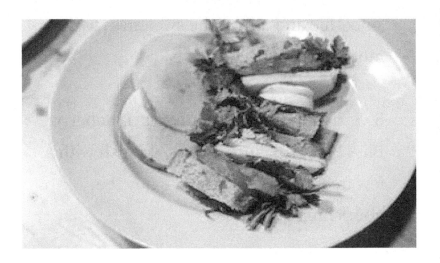

Ingredients:

- 2 salmon fillets (wild-caught is ideal)
- 1 lemon, thinly sliced

- 2 tablespoons fresh dill, chopped

- 2 cloves garlic, minced

- 1 tablespoon olive oil

- Salt and pepper to taste

- Lemon wedges for serving

Instructions:

1. *Preheat Oven (5 minutes):* Preheat your oven to 375°F (190°C) and line a baking sheet with parchment paper. This dish is rich in omega-3 fatty acids, which are excellent for skin health.

2. *Prepare Salmon (2 minutes):* Place the salmon filets on the prepared baking sheet.

3. *Mix Ingredients (3 minutes):* In a small bowl, combine the minced garlic, chopped fresh dill, and olive oil. These ingredients will infuse the salmon with flavor and provide anti-inflammatory benefits.

4. *Season Salmon (1 minute):* Drizzle the dill and garlic mixture evenly over the salmon filets. Season the salmon with a pinch of salt and a dash of black pepper.

5. *Add Lemon (2 minutes):* Lay thin slices of lemon on top of each filet. Lemon adds a refreshing twist and vitamin C, which promotes collagen production for skin elasticity.

6. *Wrap and Bake (15-20 minutes):*
Carefully fold the edges of the parchment
paper over the salmon, creating a packet.
This helps steam the fish, keeping it moist
and flavorful. Bake in the preheated oven for
about 15-20 minutes, or until the salmon
flakes easily with a fork. Cooking times may
vary depending on the thickness of your
salmon fillets.

7. *Serve (2 minutes):* Once done, remove the
salmon from the oven and carefully open the
parchment packets. Be cautious of the hot
steam. Serve your Baked Salmon with
Lemon and Dill with lemon wedges for an
extra burst of citrusy flavor. Enjoy this
omega-3 rich dish that's gentle on your skin
and delightful to your taste buds!

These time frames are approximate and can vary based on your familiarity with the recipes and cooking equipment. Enjoy your skin-nourishing culinary creations!

RECIPE 3:

Spinach and Avocado Salad

Total Time: Approximately 15 minutes

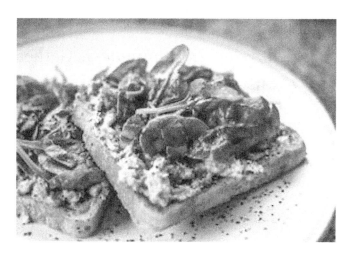

Ingredients:

- 2 cups fresh spinach leaves
- 1 ripe avocado, sliced
- 1/4 cup sliced almonds

- 1/4 cup crumbled feta cheese (optional)
- 2 tablespoons extra-virgin olive oil
- 1 tablespoon balsamic vinegar
- Salt and pepper to taste

Instructions:

1. *Prepare Ingredients (5 minutes):* Gather all your ingredients and equipment.

2. *Assemble Salad (5 minutes):* In a large salad bowl, combine the fresh spinach leaves, sliced avocado, sliced almonds, and crumbled feta cheese (if using). These ingredients provide a nutrient-packed punch for your skin.

3. *Prepare Dressing (2 minutes):* In a separate small bowl, whisk together the extra-virgin olive oil and balsamic vinegar. Season with salt and pepper to taste.

4. *Toss (2 minutes):* Drizzle the dressing over the salad ingredients and gently toss until everything is well coated.

5. *Serve (1 minute):* Divide the salad into individual serving plates or bowls. Enjoy the fresh and skin-loving flavors!

RECIPE 4:

Creamy Sweet Potato Soup

Total Time: Approximately 40 minutes

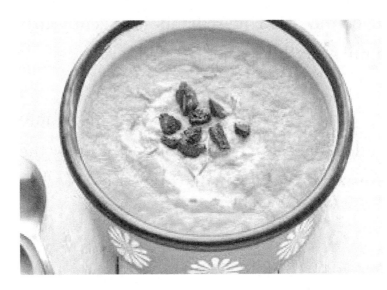

Ingredients:

- 2 large sweet potatoes, peeled and diced
- 1 onion, chopped

- 2 cloves garlic, minced

- 4 cups vegetable broth

- 1/2 cup coconut milk

- 1 teaspoon ground ginger

- Salt and pepper to taste

- Fresh cilantro leaves for garnish (optional)

Instructions:

1. *Preparation (10 minutes):* Gather all your ingredients and equipment.

2. *Saute (5 minutes):* In a large pot, sauté the chopped onion and minced garlic in a bit of olive oil until they become fragrant and translucent.

3. *Add Sweet Potatoes (5 minutes):* Add the diced sweet potatoes to the pot and sauté for another 5 minutes, stirring occasionally.

4. *Add Broth and Simmer (15 minutes):* Pour in the vegetable broth and bring the mixture to a boil. Reduce heat, cover, and simmer for about 15 minutes, or until the sweet potatoes are tender.

5. *Blend (2 minutes):* Use an immersion blender or transfer the soup to a blender in batches to puree until smooth and creamy.

6. *Add Coconut Milk (2 minutes):* Return the soup to the pot, add the coconut milk, and stir well. Season with ground ginger,

salt, and pepper to taste. Simmer for an additional 5 minutes.

7. *Serve (1 minute):* Ladle the creamy sweet potato soup into bowls, garnish with fresh cilantro leaves if desired, and savor the comforting flavors.

Recipe 5:

Lemon-Grilled Chicken Skewers

Total Time: Approximately 30 minutes

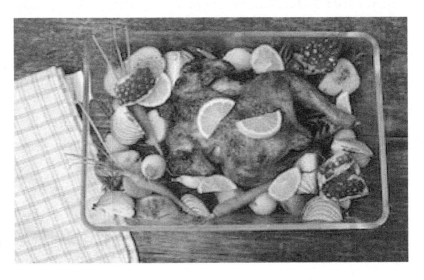

Ingredients:

- 2 boneless, skinless chicken breasts, cut into cubes

- Zest and juice of 1 lemon

- 2 cloves garlic, minced

- 1 tablespoon fresh rosemary, chopped

- 2 tablespoons olive oil

- Salt and pepper to taste

- Wooden skewers, soaked in water for 30 minutes

Instructions:

1. *Preparation (5 minutes):* Gather all your ingredients and equipment.

2. *Prepare Marinade (5 minutes):* In a bowl, combine the lemon zest, lemon juice, minced garlic, chopped rosemary, olive oil, salt, and pepper. This marinade will infuse the chicken with a burst of flavor.

3. *Marinate Chicken (10 minutes):* Thread the chicken cubes onto the soaked wooden skewers. Place the skewers in a shallow dish and pour the marinade over them. Let the chicken marinate for about 10 minutes, turning occasionally.

4. *Grill (8-10 minutes):* Preheat your grill or grill pan to medium-high heat. Grill the chicken skewers for 4-5 minutes per side, or until they are cooked through and have beautiful grill marks.

5. *Serve (2 minutes):* Remove the skewers from the grill and let them rest for a minute. Serve your Lemon-Grilled Chicken Skewers

with a side of quinoa or a fresh salad for a skin-healthy meal.

RECIPE 6:

Chia Seed Pudding

Total Time: Approximately 6 hours (mostly chilling time)

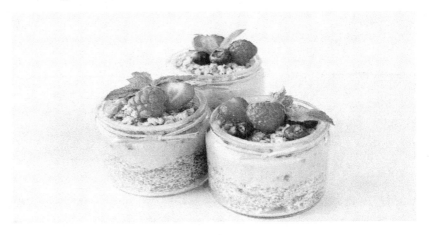

Ingredients:

- 1/4 cup chia seeds

- 1 cup unsweetened almond milk (or your preferred milk)
- 1 tablespoon honey or maple syrup (optional)
- 1/2 teaspoon vanilla extract
- Fresh berries for topping

Instructions:

1. *Preparation (5 minutes):* Gather all your ingredients and equipment.

2. *Mix (1 minute):* In a bowl, combine the chia seeds, unsweetened almond milk, honey or maple syrup (if desired), and vanilla extract. Chia seeds are a great source

of omega-3s and add a delightful texture to this pudding.

3. *Stir (1 minute):* Stir the mixture well, making sure the chia seeds are evenly distributed. Cover the bowl and refrigerate for at least 6 hours or overnight. You can give it a stir after an hour to prevent clumping.

4. *Serve (1 minute):* When ready to serve, spoon the Chia Seed Pudding into serving bowls or jars, and top with fresh berries. This pudding is not only delicious but also hydrating for your skin.

RECIPE 7:

Roasted Beet and Goat Cheese Salad

Total Time: Approximately 50 minutes

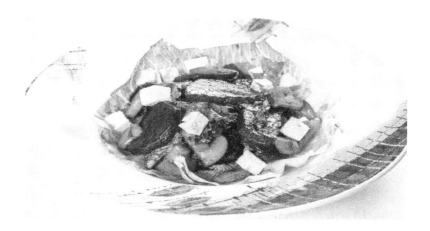

Ingredients:

- 3 medium-sized beets, peeled and cubed

- 2 cups mixed greens (e.g., arugula, spinach, or kale)
- 1/4 cup crumbled goat cheese
- 1/4 cup walnuts, toasted and chopped
- 2 tablespoons extra-virgin olive oil
- 1 tablespoon balsamic vinegar
- Salt and pepper to taste

Instructions:

1. *Preparation (10 minutes):* Gather all your ingredients and equipment.

2. *Roast Beets (40 minutes):* Preheat your oven to 400°F (200°C). Place the cubed beets on a baking sheet, drizzle with a bit of

olive oil, and season with salt and pepper. Roast for about 35-40 minutes or until the beets are tender. Let them cool.

3. *Assemble Salad (5 minutes):* In a salad bowl, combine the mixed greens, roasted beets, crumbled goat cheese, and toasted chopped walnuts.

4. *Prepare Dressing (2 minutes):* In a small bowl, whisk together the extra-virgin olive oil and balsamic vinegar. Season with salt and pepper.

5. *Dress Salad (1 minute):* Drizzle the dressing over the salad ingredients and toss gently to coat. Serve your Roasted Beet and

Goat Cheese Salad as a colorful and skin-loving dish.

RECIPE 8:

Turmeric and Ginger Tea

Total Time: Approximately 15 minutes

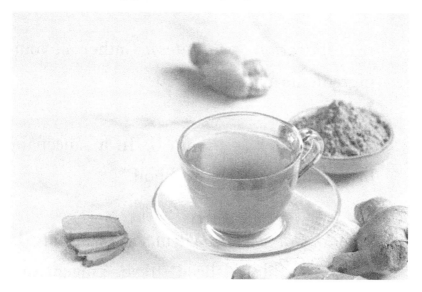

Ingredients:

- 2 cups water

- 1-inch piece of fresh ginger, thinly sliced

- 1 teaspoon ground turmeric

- 1 tablespoon honey (optional)

Instructions:

1. *Preparation (5 minutes):* Gather all your ingredients and equipment.

2. *Boil Water (5 minutes):* In a saucepan, bring 2 cups of water to a boil.

3. *Add Ginger and Turmeric (5 minutes):* Add the thinly sliced fresh ginger and ground turmeric to the boiling water. Reduce the heat and simmer for about 5 minutes.

4. *Strain and Sweeten (1 minute):* Remove the saucepan from the heat and strain the tea into cups. If desired, sweeten with honey for a touch of sweetness and enjoy the soothing and anti-inflammatory benefits of Turmeric and Ginger Tea.

RECIPE 9:

Citrus Grilled Shrimp

Total Time: Approximately 20 minutes

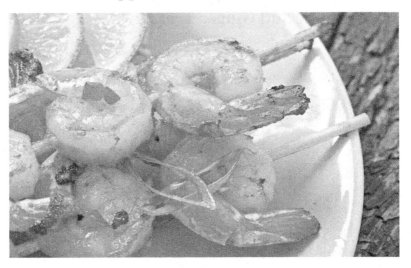

Ingredients:

- 1 pound large shrimp, peeled and deveined
- Zest and juice of 1 lemon

- Zest and juice of 1 lime
- 2 cloves garlic, minced
- 2 tablespoons olive oil
- Fresh cilantro leaves for garnish (optional)
- Salt and pepper to taste

Instructions:

1. *Preparation (5 minutes):* Gather all your ingredients and equipment.

2. *Marinate Shrimp (10 minutes):* In a bowl, combine the peeled and deveined shrimp with the lemon zest, lime zest, lemon juice, lime juice, minced garlic, olive oil, salt, and pepper. Allow the shrimp to marinate for about 10 minutes.

3. *Grill (5 minutes):* Preheat your grill or grill pan to medium-high heat. Grill the marinated shrimp for about 2-3 minutes per side or until they turn pink and are cooked through.

4. *Serve (1 minute):* Remove the grilled shrimp from the heat and garnish with fresh cilantro leaves if desired. Enjoy the zesty and skin-loving flavors of Citrus Grilled Shrimp.

RECIPE 10:

Coconut and Mango Chia Pudding

Total Time: Approximately 6 hours (mostly chilling time)

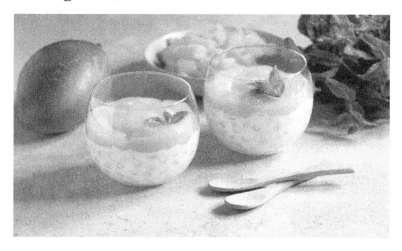

Ingredients:

- 1/4 cup chia seeds
- 1 cup coconut milk (canned or carton)

- 1 ripe mango, diced

- 1 tablespoon honey (optional)

- Unsweetened shredded coconut for topping

Instructions:

1. *Preparation (5 minutes):* Gather all your ingredients and equipment.

2. *Mix (1 minute):* In a bowl, combine the chia seeds and coconut milk. Stir well to evenly distribute the chia seeds.

3. *Chill (6 hours or more):* Cover the bowl and refrigerate for at least 6 hours or overnight, allowing the chia seeds to absorb the coconut milk and thicken.

4. *Assemble (2 minutes):* When ready to serve, spoon the Coconut and Mango Chia Pudding into serving glasses or jars. Top with diced ripe mango, a drizzle of honey if desired, and a sprinkle of unsweetened shredded coconut for a tropical and skin-loving treat.

RECIPE 11:

Total Time: Approximately 15 minutes

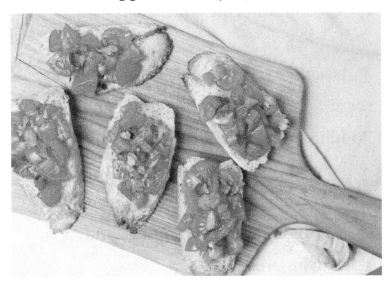

Ingredients:

- 4 ripe tomatoes, diced
- 2 cloves garlic, minced
- 1/4 cup fresh basil leaves, chopped

- 2 tablespoons extra-virgin olive oil
- 1 tablespoon balsamic vinegar
- Salt and pepper to taste
- Whole-grain baguette slices, toasted

Instructions:

1. *Preparation (5 minutes):* Gather all your ingredients and equipment.

2. *Mix Ingredients (5 minutes):* In a bowl, combine the diced tomatoes, minced garlic, chopped fresh basil, extra-virgin olive oil, balsamic vinegar, salt, and pepper. This vibrant mixture is rich in antioxidants and flavor.

3. *Toast Baguette (5 minutes):* Toast the whole-grain baguette slices until they're lightly crisp.

4. *Serve (1 minute):* Top the toasted baguette slices with the tomato and basil mixture. Drizzle with a bit of extra olive oil if desired. Enjoy your Tomato and Basil Bruschetta as a flavorful and skin-friendly appetizer.

RECIPE 12:

Lemon-Herb Baked Cod

Total Time: Approximately 25 minutes

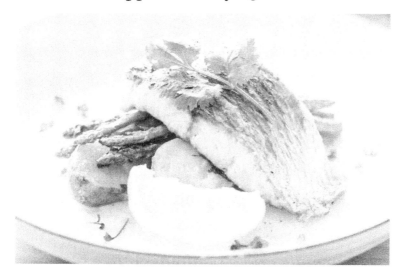

Ingredients:

- 2 cod fillets
- Zest and juice of 1 lemon

- 2 cloves garlic, minced

- 2 tablespoons fresh parsley, chopped

- 2 tablespoons fresh dill, chopped

- 2 tablespoons olive oil

- Salt and pepper to taste

- Lemon wedges for serving

Instructions:

1. *Preparation (10 minutes):* Gather all your ingredients and equipment.

2. *Marinate Cod (10 minutes):* In a bowl, combine the lemon zest, lemon juice, minced garlic, chopped fresh parsley, chopped fresh dill, olive oil, salt, and

pepper. Marinate the cod fillets in this mixture for about 10 minutes.

3. *Bake (15 minutes):* Preheat your oven to 375°F (190°C). Place the marinated cod fillets on a baking sheet. Bake for about 12-15 minutes or until the cod flakes easily with a fork.

4. *Serve (1 minute):* Remove the baked cod from the oven, garnish with lemon wedges, and savor the fresh and zesty flavors of Lemon-Herb Baked Cod.

RECIPE 13:

Mixed Berry Parfait

Total Time: Approximately 10 minutes

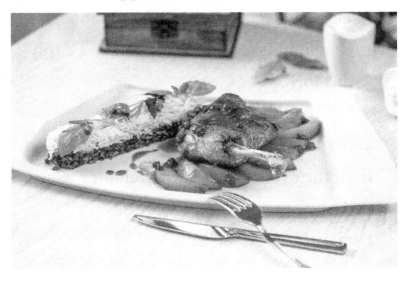

Ingredients:

- 1 cup mixed berries (e.g., strawberries, blueberries, raspberries)

- 1 cup Greek yogurt (or dairy-free alternative)
- 1/2 cup granola
- 1 tablespoon honey (optional)

Instructions:

1. *Preparation (5 minutes):* Gather all your ingredients and equipment.

2. *Layer (5 minutes):* In a glass or parfait dish, start with a layer of Greek yogurt. Add a layer of mixed berries, then a layer of granola. Repeat the layers until the glass is filled.

3. *Drizzle (1 minute):* Drizzle honey over the top layer if desired, for a touch of sweetness.

4. *Enjoy (1 minute):* Dig in and enjoy your Mixed Berry Parfait as a delicious and skin-nourishing breakfast or snack.

Recipe 14:

Broccoli and Almond Salad

Total Time: Approximately 20 minutes

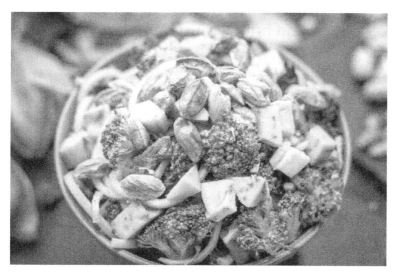

Ingredients:

- 2 cups fresh broccoli florets
- 1/4 cup sliced almonds, toasted

- 1/4 cup dried cranberries

- 2 tablespoons red onion, finely chopped

- 2 tablespoons Greek yogurt (or dairy-free alternative)

- 1 tablespoon apple cider vinegar

- 1 teaspoon honey (optional)

- Salt and pepper to taste

Instructions:

1. *Preparation (10 minutes):* Gather all your ingredients and equipment.

2. *Blanch Broccoli (5 minutes):* In a pot of boiling water, blanch the fresh broccoli florets for about 2-3 minutes until they're bright green and slightly tender.

Immediately transfer them to an ice bath to stop the cooking process. Drain well.

3. *Toast Almonds (3 minutes):* In a dry skillet, toast the sliced almonds over medium heat until they turn golden brown and fragrant.

4. *Mix Dressing (2 minutes):* In a small bowl, whisk together the Greek yogurt, apple cider vinegar, honey (if using), salt, and pepper to create the dressing.

5. *Assemble Salad (2 minutes):* In a salad bowl, combine the blanched broccoli florets, toasted sliced almonds, dried cranberries, and finely chopped red onion. Drizzle the

dressing over the salad and toss gently to coat.

6. *Serve (1 minute):* Serve your Broccoli and Almond Salad as a crunchy and flavorful side dish or light lunch.

RECIPE 15:

Papaya and Pineapple Smoothie

Total Time: Approximately 10 minutes

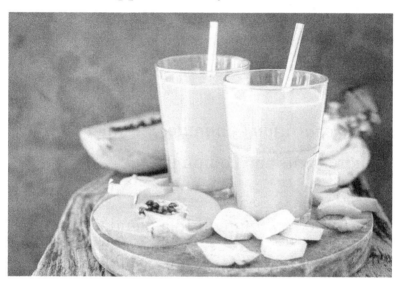

Ingredients:

- 1 cup fresh papaya, diced
- 1/2 cup fresh pineapple chunks

- 1/2 cup coconut water
- 1/2 cup Greek yogurt (or dairy-free alternative)
- 1 tablespoon honey (optional)
- Ice cubes (optional)

Instructions:

1. *Preparation (5 minutes):* Gather all your ingredients and equipment.

2. *Blend (3 minutes):* In a blender, combine the fresh papaya, fresh pineapple chunks, coconut water, Greek yogurt (or dairy-free alternative), and honey if desired. Add ice cubes if you prefer a colder smoothie.

3. *Blend until smooth and creamy.*

4. *Serve (2 minutes):* Pour your Papaya and Pineapple Smoothie into a glass and enjoy the tropical and skin-loving flavors. This smoothie is rich in vitamins and hydration, making it a refreshing choice.

10- Day Dietary Plan For Shingles & Psoriasis Warriors

This plan includes a variety of skin-nourishing recipes to promote skin health:

Day 1: *Skin-Glowing Start*

Breakfast: Blueberry Bliss Smoothie
- A refreshing and antioxidant-rich smoothie to kickstart your day.

Lunch: Spinach and Avocado Salad
- Packed with vitamins and healthy fats for radiant skin.

Dinner: Lemon-Grilled Chicken Skewers

- A protein-packed dinner with a zesty twist.

Day 2: *Superfood Delights*

Breakfast: Chia Seed Pudding
- A fiber-rich breakfast loaded with omega-3s for skin health.

Lunch: Quinoa and Roasted Vegetable Bowl
- A balanced meal featuring quinoa and colorful veggies.

Dinner: Creamy Sweet Potato Soup
- Comforting and rich in skin-loving beta-carotene.

Day 3: *Refresh and Rehydrate*

Breakfast: Cucumber and Mint Infused
Water
- A hydrating and refreshing start to your
day.

Lunch: Tomato and Basil Bruschetta
- A light and flavorful appetizer.

Dinner: Mixed Berry Parfait
- A delightful parfait with yogurt and fresh
berries.

Day 4: *Skin-Boosting Goodness*

Breakfast: Oatmeal with Berries and Almonds
- Nutrient-rich oats and antioxidants from berries.

Lunch: Coconut and Mango Chia Pudding
- A tropical chia seed pudding for a midday treat.

Dinner: Citrus Grilled Shrimp
- A zesty and protein-packed dinner option.

Day 5: Veggie-Packed Finale

Breakfast: Papaya and Pineapple Smoothie
- A tropical and vitamin C-rich smoothie.

Lunch: Broccoli and Almond Salad
- A crunchy and nutritious salad.

Dinner: Grilled Vegetable and Quinoa Stuffed Bell Peppers
- A satisfying and colorful end to your 5-day plan.

Day 6: Radiant Skin Kickoff

Breakfast: Banana and Almond Butter Smoothie Bowl
- A creamy and nutritious breakfast bowl to start your day.

Lunch: Grilled Asparagus with Lemon Zest
- A simple yet flavorful side dish that's gentle on the skin.

Dinner: Baked Salmon with Lemon and Dill
- Omega-3-rich salmon for skin health.

Day 7: Nutrient-Packed Meals

Breakfast: Chia Seed Pudding
- A fiber and omega-3-rich pudding for a satisfying start.

Lunch: Roasted Beet and Goat Cheese Salad
- A vibrant salad packed with antioxidants.

Dinner: Turmeric and Ginger Tea (Serve with a light salad)
- A soothing and anti-inflammatory tea with a refreshing salad.

Day 8: Flavorful and Hydrating

Breakfast: Coconut and Mango Chia Pudding
- A tropical chia seed pudding to brighten your morning.

Lunch: Spinach and Avocado Salad
- A nutrient-dense salad for glowing skin.

Dinner: Tomato and Basil Bruschetta (Serve with a side of grilled vegetables)
- A light and flavorful appetizer paired with veggies for a balanced meal.

Day 9: Omega-3 Power

Breakfast: Oatmeal with Berries and Almonds
- A fiber and antioxidant-rich breakfast to fuel your day.

Lunch: Lemon-Herb Baked Cod
- Zesty baked cod for skin health.

Dinner: Quinoa and Roasted Vegetable Bowl
- A hearty and colorful bowl packed with nutrients.

Day 10: A Vibrant Finale

Breakfast: Papaya and Pineapple Smoothie
- A tropical and vitamin C-rich smoothie.

Lunch: Broccoli and Almond Salad
- A crunchy salad with skin-loving almonds.

Dinner: Mixed Berry Parfait
- A delightful parfait with yogurt and fresh berries.

As always, adjust portion sizes and ingredients to suit your preferences and dietary needs. Don't forget to drink plenty of water throughout the day to stay hydrated and support healthy skin.

Health Tips To Fight Shingles and Psoriasis

Here are some effective health tips to help you in your battle against these conditions:

1. Seek Support and Understanding

You are not alone in this fight. Reach out to friends, family, or support groups to share your journey. Seek understanding and empathy, because emotional well-being is integral to healing.

2. Consult a Skilled Dermatologist

Find a dermatologist experienced in treating psoriasis. They can provide personalized treatment plans, monitor your progress, and offer guidance tailored to your specific condition.

3. Embrace a Mind-Body Connection

Practice relaxation techniques such as meditation, yoga, or deep breathing exercises. Stress can exacerbate shingles and psoriasis, so nurturing your mental health is vital.

4. Prioritize Nutrition

As mentioned earlier, nourishing your body with skin-friendly foods is crucial. A balanced diet rich in antioxidants, omega-3 fatty acids, and vitamins can aid in managing symptoms.

5. Stay Hydrated

Keep your body and skin hydrated. Drink plenty of water to maintain skin elasticity and support its natural barrier function.

6. Gentle Skin Care

Use mild, fragrance-free skincare products. Avoid harsh soaps and opt for gentle cleansers and moisturizers. Pat your skin dry instead of rubbing it.

7. Medication Adherence

If your dermatologist prescribes medication, follow their instructions diligently. Consistency is key in managing flare-ups.

8. UV Therapy

Consider phototherapy, under the guidance of a medical professional. Controlled exposure to ultraviolet (UV) light can help alleviate psoriasis symptoms.

9. Avoid Triggers

Identify and avoid triggers that worsen your symptoms. These may include stress, certain foods, or environmental factors.

10. Protect Your Skin

Shield your skin from extreme weather conditions. Use sunscreen to protect against sunburn, which can trigger psoriasis outbreaks.

11. Be Patient and Kind to Yourself

Healing takes time. Understand that both shingles and psoriasis are chronic conditions, and there will be ups and downs. Treat yourself with patience and self-compassion.

12. Monitor Your Skin

Regularly inspect your skin for changes or flare-ups. Being vigilant allows you to catch and address issues early.

13. Share Your Experience

Share your journey with others. You might inspire and offer hope to someone else battling the same conditions.

14. Embrace Positivity

Cultivate a positive mindset. Surround yourself with activities and people that uplift you. A positive outlook can have a profound impact on your overall health.

15. Celebrate Small Victories

Celebrate every small victory, whether it's a day without discomfort or a noticeable improvement. Each step forward is worth acknowledging.

16. Consult Your Healthcare Team

Stay in close contact with your healthcare team. They can adjust your treatment plan as needed and offer valuable advice.

Remember, your health journey is unique, and there is no one-size-fits-all solution. These tips are meant to provide guidance and support, but it's essential to work closely with your healthcare providers to find the best path forward for your specific condition. You are a warrior, and with patience and determination, you can manage and thrive despite the challenges of shingles and psoriasis.

Preventive Measures For Shingles

1. Vaccination (Shingrix): If you're over the age of 50, consider getting the Shingrix vaccine. It significantly reduces the risk of developing shingles and can also help reduce the severity of the illness if you do contract it.

2. Boost Your Immune System: A strong immune system can help prevent shingles. Maintain a healthy lifestyle with regular exercise, balanced nutrition, and sufficient sleep.

3. Stress Management: Chronic stress can weaken your immune system, increasing the risk of shingles. Practice stress-reduction techniques like meditation, yoga, or deep breathing exercises.

4. Hand Hygiene: Good hand hygiene can prevent the spread of the varicella-zoster virus, which causes shingles. Wash your hands regularly, especially if you've been in contact with someone who has shingles.

5. Avoid Close Contact: If you have shingles, avoid close contact with individuals who haven't had chickenpox or the vaccine, as they can contract chickenpox from you.

Preventive Measures for Psoriasis

1. Maintain a Healthy Diet: Consuming a balanced diet rich in fruits, vegetables, whole grains, and lean proteins can help manage psoriasis. Some individuals find that avoiding trigger foods, such as processed foods, red meat, and dairy, helps reduce flare-ups.

2. Stay Hydrated: Proper hydration supports skin health. Drinking enough water can help maintain skin elasticity and minimize dryness.

3. Avoid Skin Trauma: Be gentle with your skin. Avoid scratching, picking, or scrubbing your skin vigorously, as this can worsen psoriasis symptoms.

4. Sun Protection: While some sunlight can benefit psoriasis, excessive sun exposure can trigger flare-ups. Use sunscreen and limit your time in direct sunlight.

5. Manage Stress: Stress is a known trigger for psoriasis. Engage in stress-reduction activities like yoga, meditation, or hobbies you enjoy.

6. Alcohol and Smoking: Limit alcohol consumption and avoid smoking, as both can exacerbate psoriasis symptoms.

7. Medication Adherence: If you're prescribed medication for psoriasis, take it as directed by your healthcare provider. Consistency is vital in managing the condition.

8. Moisturize: Keep your skin well-moisturized with fragrance-free moisturizers. This helps alleviate dryness and itching associated with psoriasis.

9. Regular Check-Ups: Regularly see your dermatologist for check-ups, even when your psoriasis is in remission. Early detection and intervention can prevent severe flare-ups.

10. Lifestyle Choices: Maintain a healthy lifestyle with adequate sleep, regular exercise, and proper stress management. A balanced life contributes to overall well-being and can help manage psoriasis.

Remember that shingles and psoriasis are complex conditions, and what works for one person may not work for another. It's essential to work closely with healthcare professionals to develop a personalized prevention and management plan tailored to your specific needs. By taking proactive measures and making healthy choices, you can reduce the risk of these conditions and enjoy better skin health.

CONCLUSION

In closing, my fellow warriors for skin health, this cookbook isn't just about recipes; it's a testament to your strength and resilience. It's a reminder that even in the face of shingles and psoriasis, you have the power to nourish, heal, and thrive.

Throughout these pages, we've embarked on a flavorful journey, embracing the connection between what we put on our plates and how it impacts our skin. We've celebrated the vibrancy of fruits and vegetables, the comfort of hearty soups, and the joy of savoring every bite. Each recipe has been a small victory a step towards healthier, happier skin.

But remember, this cookbook is more than just a collection of ingredients and instructions; it's a companion on your path to wellness. It's a friend cheering you on when flare-ups try to dim your spirit. It's a partner in the kitchen, reminding you that every meal you create is a declaration of self-love.

As you continue your journey, may these recipes not only nourish your skin but also nurture your soul. May every meal be a moment of self-care, a celebration of your resilience, and a testament to your unwavering spirit.

You are more than your skin conditions; you are warriors, and this cookbook is your shield against adversity. Together, we stand strong, united by the belief that healing begins on the plate. Keep cooking, keep savoring, and keep shining. Your radiant skin is a testament to your inner strength, your self-love, and your unwavering determination to live your best life.

GLOSSARY

1. Antioxidants: Compounds found in foods like berries, tomatoes, and leafy greens that protect the skin from damage caused by free radicals, promoting skin health.

2. Omega-3 Fatty Acids: Essential fats, commonly found in salmon, flaxseeds, and walnuts, known for their anti-inflammatory properties and their potential to alleviate skin conditions.

3. Gluten-Free: A diet that excludes gluten, a protein found in wheat, barley, and rye. Some individuals with psoriasis find relief from symptoms on a gluten-free diet.

4. Immune System: The body's defense mechanism that fights infections and diseases. A strong immune system is essential for preventing and managing shingles and psoriasis.

5. Inflammation: The body's natural response to injury or infection. Chronic inflammation can exacerbate skin conditions like psoriasis.

6. Meditation: A mindfulness practice that reduces stress and promotes relaxation, benefiting skin health.

7. Phototherapy: A medical treatment involving controlled exposure to ultraviolet

(UV) light, sometimes used to manage psoriasis symptoms.

8. Psoriasis Plaque: Raised, reddish patches of skin covered with a silvery-white scale, a hallmark symptom of psoriasis.

9. Stress Reduction: Techniques like meditation, yoga, and deep breathing exercises that help lower stress levels, which can trigger or worsen skin conditions.

10. Topical Treatment: Medications or creams applied directly to the skin to manage psoriasis symptoms.

11. Varicella-Zoster Virus: The virus responsible for both chickenpox and shingles. Reactivation of this virus causes shingles.

12. Whole Foods: Unprocessed or minimally processed foods that retain their natural nutrients, such as fruits, vegetables, whole grains, and lean proteins.

13. Omega-3 Supplements: Capsules or oils containing omega-3 fatty acids, sometimes used as a dietary supplement to manage skin conditions.

14. Moisturizer: Skincare product used to hydrate and protect the skin, especially important for individuals with psoriasis to prevent dryness and itching.

15. Biologics: A type of medication used to treat severe psoriasis by targeting specific parts of the immune system.

16. Gluten Sensitivity: A condition where the body reacts negatively to gluten, though it falls short of celiac disease. Some individuals with psoriasis may benefit from a gluten-free diet.

17. UVB Therapy: A form of phototherapy using UVB light to manage psoriasis symptoms.

18. Gluten-Free Flours: Alternative flours made from grains like rice, almond, or coconut, suitable for gluten-free diets.

19. Autoimmune Disease: Conditions where the immune system mistakenly attacks healthy cells in the body, as seen in psoriasis.

20. Immune-Boosting Foods: Foods like citrus fruits, garlic, and spinach that support a healthy immune system.

Made in United States
Orlando, FL
18 July 2025

63082131R00056